Hair

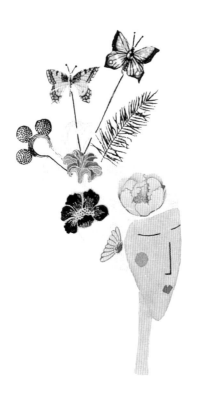

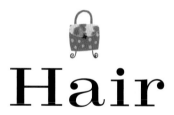

Hair

100 styling secrets

Carol Morley & Liz Wilde

Time Warner Books

WARNER BOOKS

An AOL Time Warner Company

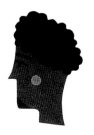
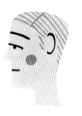
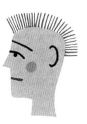
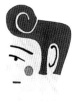

introduction

Ever been frustrated by your hair? Ever have times when you just can't get it to behave the way you want it to? Well wave goodbye to bad hair days, because this little book is crammed with 100 top tips guaranteed to get your hair into "cover girl" condition! Learn the secrets of nutrition to make your hair healthy from the inside out; discover how to seal in shine, how to tame the frizzies, and how to get body into the limpest hair. Plus professional tips for sophisticated styling and recipes for homemade hair treatments, as well as fool-proof problem solvers to help you out when things have gone wrong. Beautiful hair starts here!

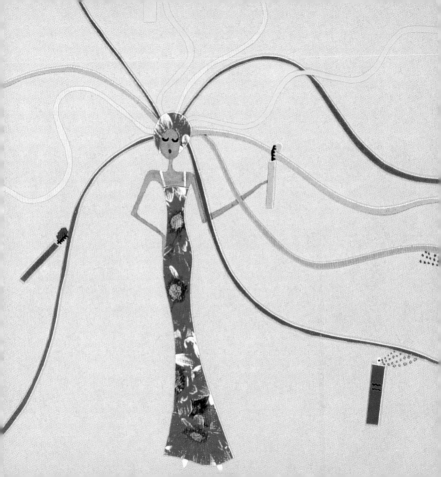

contents

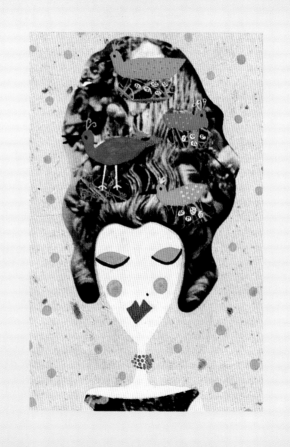

chapter 1

What the pros know

You don't need to get a head full of suds for your shampoo to do its job. Loads of lather doesn't mean cleaner hair. The amount of lather you get depends on the level of foam boosters in a shampoo, and too many can make the detergent hard on your hair. You need just enough lather to gently lift off dirt so it can be easily rinsed away—too much and you'll be in the shower twice as long!

Experts believe that most hair problems are caused by bad washing. One of the worst things you can do is to rinse away shampoo by dunking your head in soapy bathwater or by pouring over a few cups of clean water. To work right, most shampoo and conditioners need plenty of water to remove dirt and release their conditioning ingredients. So, if you don't already do so, make sure you use your spray attachment!

Heard the one about hair getting used to a shampoo? Don't believe it. Shampoo sellers use this myth to get you to change your brand, but the same shampoo will give you the same results. What *may* change is your hair. A perm, color, or different length will all affect the condition, so you might need to find a new shampoo to suit your new style.

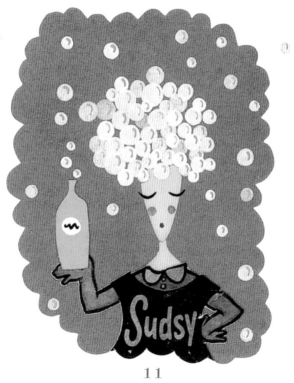

Tibet Pumpkin Oil

Soak your scalp and hair in warm olive oil for a deep conditioning. Pour a tablespoon of oil (make that two if your hair's past shoulder length) into a saucer and heat over a pan of boiling water. Massage into dry hair and then jump in the bath or shower so the heat can open up your pores and encourage the oil to sink in. After about 15 minutes, remove the oil by applying shampoo directly to your hair without rinsing first. Lather up (though you won't get many suds), then rinse and shampoo again as normal. Or try using pumpkin oil in the same way. In Tibet it is believed to be a great tonic for the hair—and the brain!

12

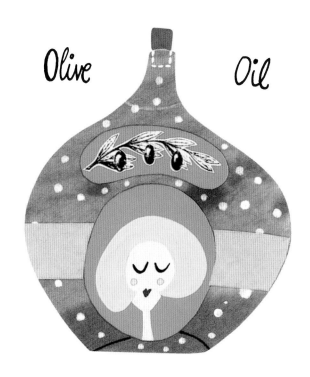

Olive Oil

5 **Hair is naturally elastic, but the more you pull it, the weaker it gets.** When your hair's wet, it loses about 25 percent of its elasticity, and overenthusiastic brushing or combing can stretch it to the breaking point. Never use a brush on wet hair, and always remove tangles with a wide-tooth comb starting from the ends and working upward. If you come across a stubborn tangle, spray it with leave-in conditioner and your comb will simply slide through.

6 **Hair experts hate 2-in-1s because it's impossible for them to do both jobs as well as a separate shampoo and conditioner can.** But that doesn't mean 2-in-1s don't come in very handy for taking down to the gym or away for the weekend when you're traveling light. Just don't make it too much of a habit.

7 **If you have long hair, give it a quick brushing before shampooing to remove any loose hairs.** The result? Your drains will get clogged less often and there will be fewer tangles for you to remove after conditioning.

8 **Feeling brave? Try giving your hair a final rinse with cold water after washing.** This closes the cuticle on each strand so that it lies flat. Presto! Instantly shiny hair.

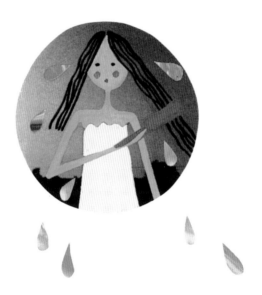

Just two days of exposure to the sun can weaken your hair by up to 50 percent, leaving it dry, discolored, and ready to break. Sit in the sun unprotected and it'll be more than just your skin that gets burned. But while you remember to smooth on a sunscreen, chances are you forget about your hair. A hat is the best defense against sun-damaged hair, but if you prefer to go bareheaded,

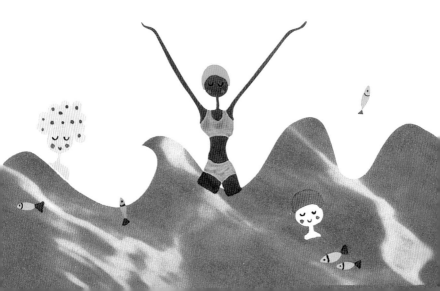

protect your locks by pouring a little high-SPF suntan lotion in with your hair spray (use oil-free lotion so it doesn't make your hair greasy). Simply squirt on before styling, and before venturing out into the sun. For protection in the pool or the sea, mix some waterproof suntan oil in with your regular conditioner and then comb through your hair, reapplying after every dip.

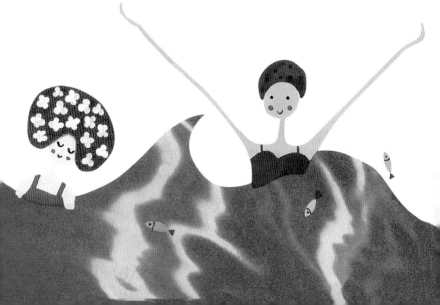

A scalp massage helps speed up the blood supply to your head, bringing all the nutrients and oxygen needed for healthy hair. Many salons offer this service, but you can easily create the same effect at home. Use your fingertips—don't scratch or rub—and work in small circular movements all over your scalp.

Panthenol is the only vitamin that can actually penetrate your hair and boost moisture levels—look for it on the labels of shampoos and conditioners. Other proteins such as collagen and elastin work by clinging to the surface of the hair to protect the cuticle, making it feel thicker.

Hair dryers can get very hot, and overuse can harm your hair. Allow your locks to dry naturally whenever possible, and never start styling until your hair's at least 80 percent dry to cut down on potential damage time. Dryers with diffuser attachments are the gentlest way to dry your hair and work well at encouraging waves.

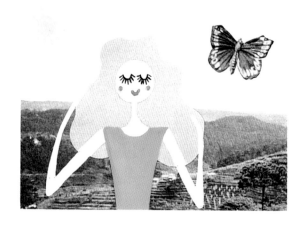

Fine hair tangles more than thick hair, curly hair tangles more than straight hair, and damaged hair tangles most of all. Instead of the cuticles lying flat, they lift up and interlock with the hairs next door (like Velcro strips). Never tug at your tangles. After shampooing, apply plenty of conditioner, then gently ease them apart. Work from the ends up with a wide-tooth comb or your fingers. Never dry your hair by rubbing with a towel—your locks will literally lock together.

A final rinse with mint tea after applying conditioner will make oily hair shine—without adding more grease.

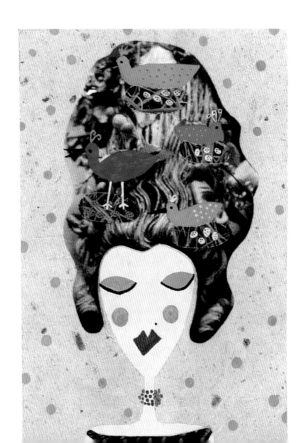

Dandruff is most common in winter as stress levels are higher and scalps sweat under hats. But those little white flakes may just mean that you're suffering from a dry scalp. Brush your hair over some dark fabric. If the flakes are small, then it's likely that your skin's dry and daily washing with a mild shampoo (look for words like "frequent use" or "baby shampoo" on the label) will clear things up. If the flakes are large, clumpy, and moist, chances are you're suffering from dandruff and need to switch to a specially formulated shampoo. Don't panic—alternate this with your regular shampoo and you should see an improvement within 2 weeks.

Experts can't decide whether product buildup actually exists, but if your hair's looking limp and lifeless, it could probably use a little help. Try this homemade deep cleanser to revitalize your locks. Pour 1 cup of white vinegar into a pan containing 5 cups of boiling water and allow the mixture to cool. Massage gently into just-washed hair. Now grit your teeth and finish with a cold-water rinse to promote shine.

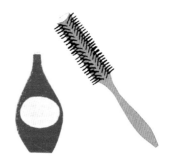

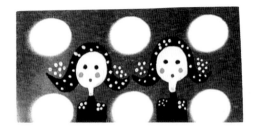

If your hair is looking dull and lack luster, try this home-made conditioning treatment: Mash one banana and mix it with 1 tablespoon of sunflower oil and $\frac{1}{2}$ tablespoon of lime juice. Spread the mixture over your hair and then cover with a plastic bag to catch any drips. Leave it in for about 30 minutes, then rinse well with warm water before shampooing.

Even oily hair needs a conditioner. All conditioners work by flattening the cuticle scales to make your hair shiny and tangle-free. Just avoid your scalp and only apply to the mid-lengths and ends.

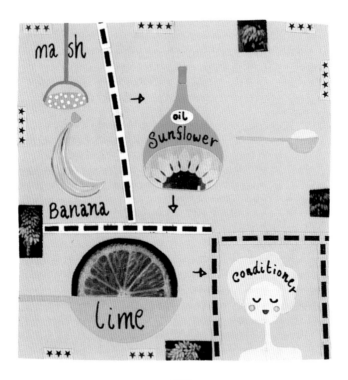

Hair is made up of almost 100 percent protein. Feed your follicles by eating protein at every meal. Fish, poultry, and meat are excellent sources of protein, as are tofu, beans, and rice. Seafood gets bonus points for providing the hair-friendly minerals iron, iodine, zinc, and selenium.

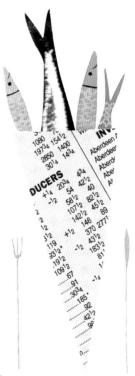

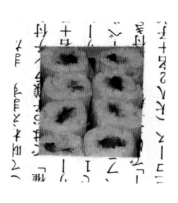

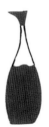

You can't expect your hair to shine if you use dirty combs and brushes. Clean them regularly in soapy water or they'll act like a magnet for all things gunky. To revive neglected hair tools, dissolve 1 tablespoon of washing soda in warm water, add a few drops of antiseptic, then swish the tools around. Tap them on the side of the sink and you'll be amazed at the dirt that dislodges. Finally, rinse in clean water and lay them on a towel to dry.

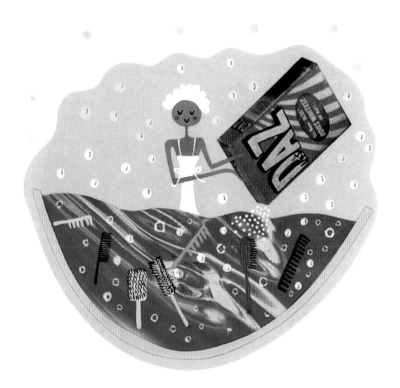

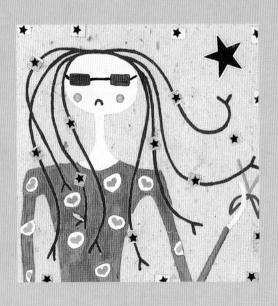

chapter 2

The right cut

The best way to find a hairstylist is by word of mouth. Ask your friends, ask your colleagues, ask anyone whose hair looks good on the street. If you can't find a non-scary salon, experiment by having your hair blow-dried before risking a cut. Check out the other customers there—most salons specialize in a certain type of clientele. If you're a trendy 25-year-old, a salon full of 60-year-old shampoo-and-sets is not likely to be the place that will transform your hair into the style of your dreams. Also, assess how helpful your hairdresser is and how comfortable he or she makes you feel. Then book that appointment.

Don't commit to a restyle without a consultation. All hairdressers should be willing to spend at least 10 minutes talking things over with you before you book that all-important first appointment. But be sure to choose a quiet moment— the middle of a busy Saturday may not be the best time for a casual chat.

Make the most of your hairstylist. During the appointment remember to ask as many questions as you can think of. You're not just paying for a cut— you're paying for your hairstylist's expertise, so make sure you get your money's worth!

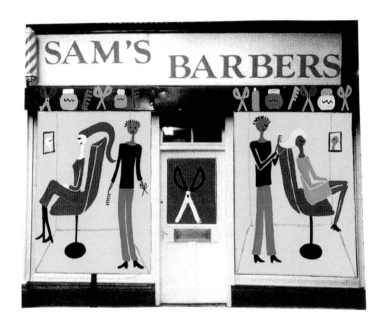

Tell your stylist how much time you plan to spend on your hair at the outset. If you're the wash-and-go type, a complicated "do" will bring you to the brink of a breakdown. And always be honest about upkeep. If you want to come in for a cut only twice a year, then be sure to say so.

A stylist should always take the time to look at your hair while it's still dry. Once you've been shampooed and your hair is wet, all the natural texture will have disappeared. If you find yourself being marched to the sink without a consultation, turn around and march straight out the door.

Taking a picture to your hairdresser is the easiest way to communicate the style you're after. But be realistic. The model probably had a stylist who spent at least 30 minutes (and sometimes up to two hours) on her hair and then stood just outside the frame, ready to tweak any unruly strands into shape. Your hair might not receive quite as much attention.

The most successful hair styles are those that suit your hair type. Trying to calm your naturally curly hair into a sleek, straight style every morning will lead to definite damage, probable tears, and an hour's less sleep.

28 **Always go to the salon looking yourself—don't make a special effort to dress up.** Wear what you usually wear and do your makeup as normal. That way the hairdresser will be able to see you as you are and help you decide on a look to suit your natural style.

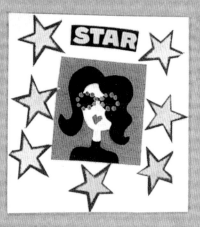

The right cut can flatter any face shape:

Long faces benefit from big, bouncy styles that add width and long, heavy bangs. Avoid flat styles and middle parts.

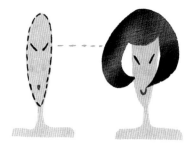

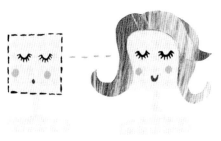

Square faces need soft, wavy styles that soften sharp angles. Avoid blunt-cut bangs and anything severe.

Round faces look best with ➡ *soft, layered cuts with face-framing bangs. Avoid too much volume and long, heavy bangs.*

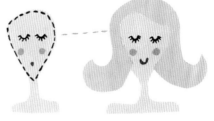

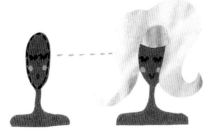

⬅ *Oval faces can wear just about any style, so make the most of your good fortune and experiment.*

Heart-shaped faces look ➡ *good with flips to balance the width at the top of the head. Avoid short cuts that frame the face.*

A good haircut can act like a face-lift—you come of out of the salon feeling like a new person. Which is why so many of us mark changes in our lives with a dramatically different cut. A new job? End of a relationship? Time to cut away the old part of you and make a fresh start.

A bad haircut is not a life sentence. On average, hair grows 6 inches a year, but however desperate you are to grow it long again, a tiny trim every two months will keep the ends healthy. What a cut won't do is make your hair grow faster. This may be the case with shaving (the more you shave, the quicker the stubble seems to appear), but your head's not a rosebush in need of pruning, and the only thing a trim will do is even out the ends to keep those splits away.

If you don't like your new style, don't panic right away. It may just take a little getting used to and an hour of experimenting with different products and drying techniques. If you're still not happy, go back to your hairstylist for some confidence-boosting and advice on how to style it. And if you're the nervous type, get your restyles done in the summer—just like a plant, your hair grows faster during the hot weather!

33 **If you're happy with your new hair style, remember to leave a tip.** Hairdressers rely on them to boost their very often meager wages, and a good tipper will be remembered at the next appointment (which means guaranteed good service). The average tip is 15 percent of the total bill for the main stylist. And don't forget to include enough extra to tip the trainee who washed your hair; this will also be gratefully received. You can be sure that his or her wages are even lower.

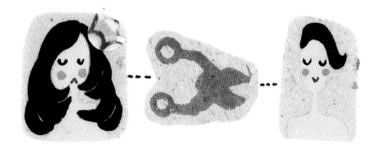

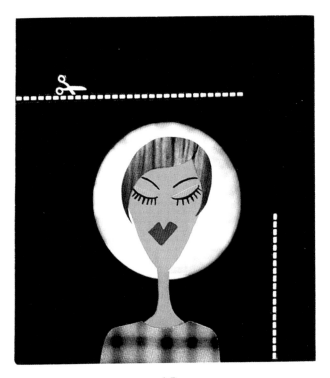

40

34 Short hair

Good:
- *It's quick and easy to care for.*
- *If your hair's fine, it'll look thicker.*
- *It will show off your face.*
- *You'll look like a new person.*
- *You may look younger.*
- *You can take risks—color mistakes grow out quickly.*

Bad:
- *You need a trim every four to six weeks to keep the shape.*
- *It's not as versatile as long hair.*

35. Long hair

Good:
- *It's very versatile.*
- *You only need a trim about every two months.*
- *Long hair softens facial flaws.*
- *You can play with it.*
- *Oh, and most men like it....*

Bad:
- *It takes longer to wash and dry.*
- *Split ends are more likely.*
- *Tangles can be a problem.*

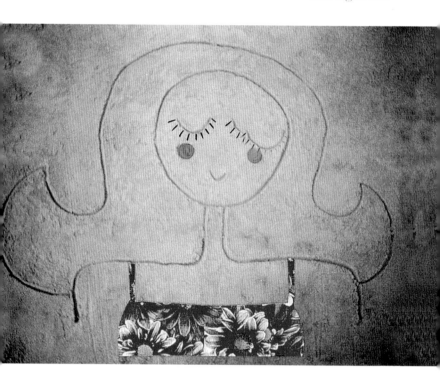

Benefits of bangs:

- Bangs disguise a high, low, or uneven hairline.
- There are at least 50 ways to style bangs, so one's got to suit you.
- Bangs are flattering as they soften facial flaws.
- Whatever style you choose, bangs will make you look younger.

A note of caution. Despite all the benefits, think long and hard before you commit. Bangs will take a long time to grow out and catch up with rest of your hair, particularly if it's long. Make sure it's really what you want before the snipping starts.

38 **Most hairstylists will be happy to trim your bangs free of charge,** but if you are feeling brave and want to give it a try yourself, here's how:

1. Clip all the rest of your hair out of the way.

2. Don't cut your bangs when your hair is wet. Your hair will shrink up by at least half an inch when it dries, leaving it shorter than you planned!

3. Carefully comb your bangs straight down and start trimming, working from the center outward.

4. Don't hold the hair down with your fingers or comb as this will alter the natural line.

5. Remember, less is more. Go slowly and comb constantly to check your line.

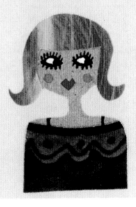

Hairdresser speak:

Layering is working from very short lengths at the nape of the neck to longer layers on top. A great body builder for fine hair but can look too bulky on thick.

Texturizing is layering that is concentrated on the ends of the hair to create texture. It works well on all hair types, especially short styles.

Razoring takes place after the basic cut is completed. Random sections are sliced out to give a softer shape. Works well on thick hair—those with fine hair should avoid it.

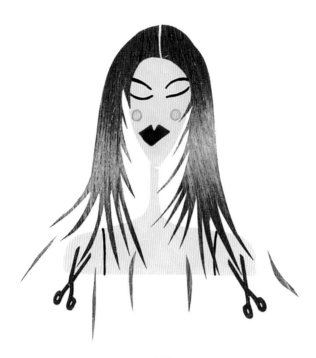

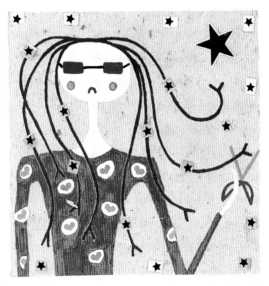

It's impossible to repair ends once they are split, so don't be tempted by products that promise to glue them back together. The results will only last until the next time you brush.

The only way to cure a case of split ends is to cut them off. For damage control, tightly twist a section of split hair: All the bad ends will stick out, ready to be snipped away.

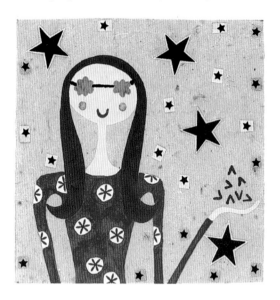

49

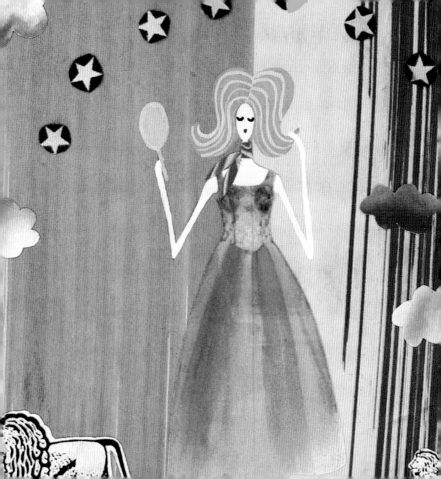

chapter 3

Coloring

41 If you want your new shade to look ultranatural, keep within your own color range. That means up to two shades lighter or darker than you are now. And don't ignore your skin tone; pale blonde hair on olive skin will always look like it came out of a bottle. As a rule, olive skin needs warm-colored hair (golden blonde, chestnut brown, etc.) and pink skin needs a cool color (caramel blonde, ash brown).

42 The biggest reason for home-coloring disappointments? Most home colorists assume that their hair will end up looking like that of the girl on the box, but it's not that simple.

Your end result depends on how your hair starts out (ie., your natural color) and anything else that's gone before. Check the color chart on the box or phone the helpline for advice before you begin. Oh, and sorry to disillusion you, but it's very likely that the model you're looking at hasn't been near a dye—let alone the one in the box she's on!

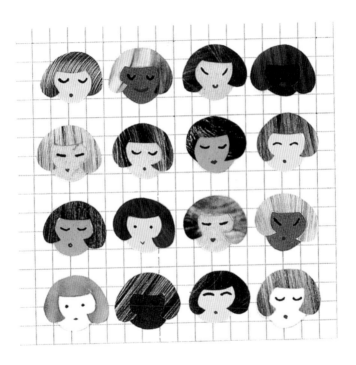

53

43   **Vegetable and plant-based colorants,** not to be mistaken for henna, which is permanent, are the best low-risk ways to dye your hair. But, as ever, there are pros and cons...

Good:
- *Can add depth, warmth, and richness to your hair color without damaging it.*
- *Will add volume and shine to fine, straight hair.*
- *Can be used to tone down or add color on top of old highlights and lowlights.*
- *Contain no chemicals so they can only improve condition.*
- *Color fades gradually so there's no chance of noticeable roots.*

Bad:
- *Lack of chemicals means they can't lighten hair.*
- *Will only last for about eight shampoos—so if you wash your hair every day your color will soon fade.*

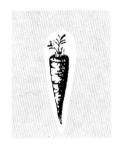

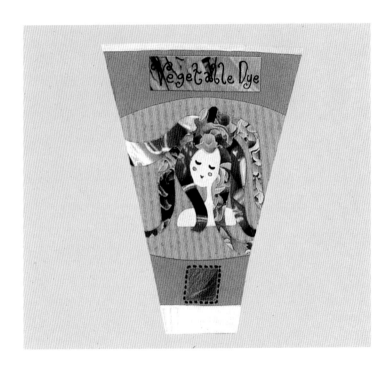

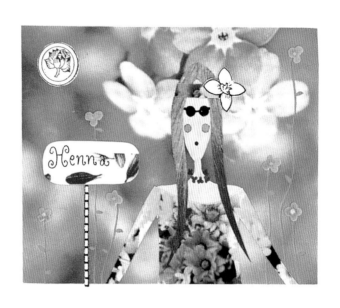

44 Looking for a natural way to color permanently? Henna has been used for thousands of years without any adverse or allergic reactions. It comes from dried plant leaves, which are crushed and made into a paste. You'll know pure henna because it smells strongly of earth, and make sure you sniff out a pure product—some herbal ones also contain chemicals to speed up the process. But just because henna is natural, don't underestimate its powers. The results will be permanent, so make sure you're going to like the color first by doing a strand test. Unlike chemical dyes, the shorter the length of time that you leave henna on, the brighter the color. Don't panic and wash too early. If you want a darker shade rather than bright red, mix about 8 ounces of strong coffee with one packet of red henna. For a richer red result, add a dash of red wine. For dry hair, add a beaten egg to the mix, and if you can't stand waiting, a squeeze of lemon juice will speed up the process.

45 There are many different shades of red to choose from (note: ruddy complexions should give this one a pass). If your skin's fair, go for any shade between strawberry blonde and vibrant red. If you're more olive-skinned, darker auburn or burgundy shades will work well on you.

Professional coloring does not come cheap, so you will want the result to last for as long as possible. To stop permanent color from fading too quickly, rinse your hair in cider vinegar before shampooing for the first two weeks after your pricey appointment.

Remember, permanent colors aren't called that for nothing! They contain chemicals that enter the hair shaft and stay there, so think carefully before you take the plunge!

When choosing your coloring expert, make sure you ask for a technician who specializes in color. He or she will have been specially trained in the use of chemicals, whereas a general hairdresser who's a jack-of-all-trades will have learned a bit about everything.

Be brutally honest about what you've put on your hair in the past. Permanent colors stay in your hair until the dye grows out (as do henna and spray-in lighteners). Your hair may still contain chemicals from a previous coloring, which will react badly with any new ones used. Keeping quiet about that dye disaster you had in your bathroom six months ago could result in a far bigger disaster happening right now.

50 **Coloring your hair means commitment.** The more dramatic the change, the faster it will need doing again. Remember, hair grows, and with it come those tell-tale roots. A permanent tint will need redoing every four weeks and highlights about every three months.

51 **When your roots are grow-ing back dark and you haven't got the time (or the money) for a salon appointment,** disguise the regrowth by applying a little dry shampoo along your part and flicking off the excess. Or use a blonde hair mascara—just don't go out in the rain!

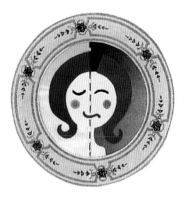

If your hair's fine, a good color job will swell the shaft and make it look thicker. Highlights are the best way to add texture and lift to limp hair, and you don't have to get your whole head done. Some slices taken from around the front will instantly brighten your face, and if you only go a few shades lighter than nature intended, upkeep will be minimal too. Which is just as well, as foil highlights don't come cheap. If you're ever offered the old-fashioned cap variety, run for your (hair's) life. Yanking pieces of hair through a thick rubber cap is hit-and-miss at best and positively painful for anyone with hair longer than shoulder length.

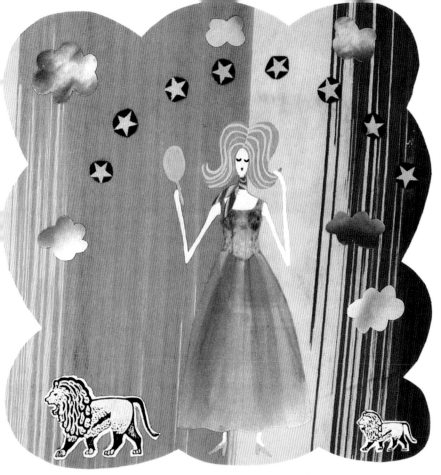

53 **Born blonde? You can look like it if you work with your own coloring.** Green or brown eyes go best with golden blonde shades, while gray- and blue-eyed types look best as ash blondes. But beware! Blonde hair is high maintenance—expect to see roots peeping through after a month. A proper bleach job is best left to the professionals, but you can lift dull hair between appointments with a post-shampoo herbal rinse. Mix 8 parts water with 1 part lemon juice, or make an infusion with 1 to 2 tablespoons of dried camomile flowers in 2 cups of boiling water. Cool and pour. Camomile can also be used to lighten hair if you want to avoid bleach. Make an infusion with 3 tablespoons of dried flowers in 12 ounces of boiling water. Add 1 teaspoon of vinegar and 4 tablespoons of lemon juice. Let cool, then pour over just-washed hair. Leave for 30 minutes.

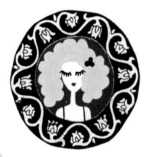

54 **If you've colored your hair darker,** sleep on an old pillowcase the first night since dark colors tend to transfer until you've shampooed again.

55 Temporary color is like makeup for hair.

The dye coats the surface and lasts until your next wash. Which is perfect for color cowards. Hair mascara lets you paint just where you want a splash of color, while sprays are best for larger sections. But be careful if you're applying the color over bleached hair: It is very porous and drinks up color. You may find that those bright pink streaks last longer than the Saturday night you intended them for.

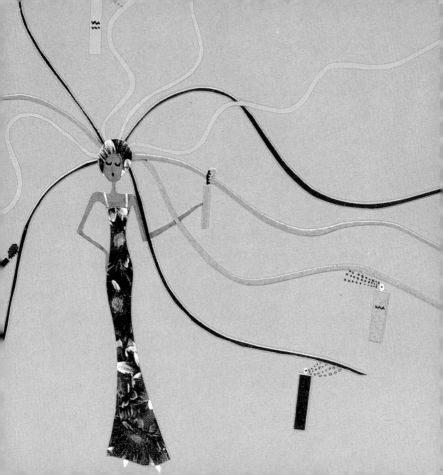

Avoid home-coloring disasters by remembering these few simple rules:

- *Any color that comes in two separate bottles and needs mixing together will last on your hair for more than a few weeks (and possibly permanently).*
- *Mix color only when you're ready to use it as it won't keep; throw out any leftover mix immediately.*
- *If you have long hair, buy two boxes of color so you don't run out.*
- *Read the instructions carefully. Most home disasters happen when you skip this step.*
- *Do a skin and strand test, it is the only way to make sure your color change will be a good one.*

- *If you're unsure about what to do, look for a helpline number on the side of the box.*

Don't like your home-done semipermanent dye? Wash your hair with a shampoo labeled "bodybuilding" or "clarifying" to deep-down clean. Alternately, soak your hair in warm olive oil for a hour (this will open up your hair's cuticle, allowing the color trapped there to be released—it will also act as a deep conditioner) then shampoo out. Done more serious damage in your bathroom? Most home color disasters can be sorted out by a professional, so put on a hat and get down to the hair salon.

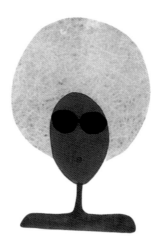

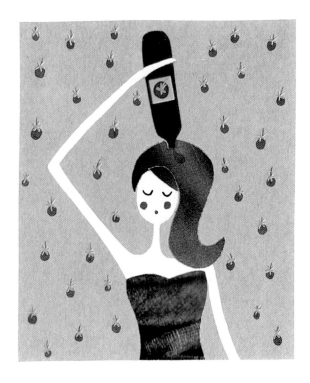

68

58 **Swimming in chlorinated pools can turn blonde hair green.** Tackle this problem by pouring either tomato juice or ketchup over your hair. Leave for 15 minutes, then shampoo out. The red food dye in the tomato will counteract the green in your hair, and the ghoulish tint will disappear.

59 **Coloring before a vacation may seem like perfect sense,** but you'll have to be extra careful to protect your hair. Keep it out of the sun or wear a hat (oxidation will fade your new color), and stay out of the ocean and chlorinated swimming pools for at least 48 hours after dyeing. The chemical process involved in coloring opens the hair's cuticle, leaving it vulnerable to damage and discoloration.

When home dyeing has left you with stained skin, dip a damp cotton ball in either baby oil, lemon juice, or perfume and gently wipe the affected area. Avoid stains in the future by smoothing a layer of petroleum jelly around your hairline before covering your hair with color.

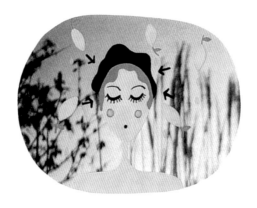

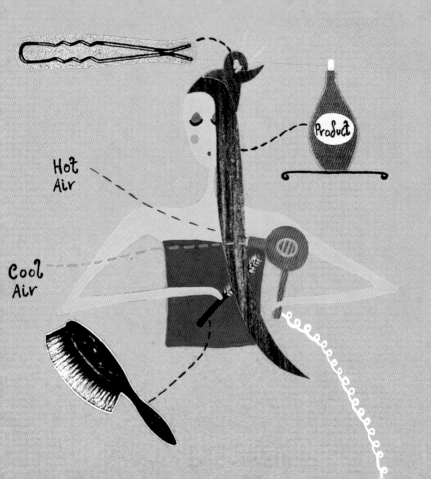

Hot
Air

Cool
Air

Product

chapter 4

Styling solutions

Choose the right tools for the job:

Brushes:
There are two types of bristles—natural and nylon. Professionals prefer natural as they have a smoothing effect on the hair and help distribute the natural oils for added shine. They're also less likely to encourage static, but some can be stiff and sharp when new. Copy a hairdresser trick and turn your just-bought brush into an old faithful by soaking the bristles in boiling water to soften them. You can use cheaper, nylon-bristle brushes, but look for ones with rounded ends so they don't scratch your scalp.

Round brushes come in many sizes, so choose one that suits your hair length (too small on long hair and you'll get yourself in a tangle). As a general rule, the brush should be big enough for your hair to wrap around more than twice. Use round brushes to style in curls and volume or to straighten kinks.

Paddle brushes are the biggest brushes around; used by hair-dressers to groom long hair without snagging.

Vent brushes are the best for blow-drying: This brush has widely spaced bristles and holes in the back so air can flow through and cut styling time. Perfect for natural styles but won't have enough fight for smoothing out frizz.

Flat brushes have bristles just on one side set on a rubber cushion. Use as a general grooming tool, but invest in something more specific for special styling.

Combs:
Tail combs have closely spaced teeth (good for teasing) and a long end for sectioning.

Wide tooth combs are invaluable for detangling wet hair without damage but no good for styling.

Pick combs have big, fat teeth for easing through tightly-curled hair.

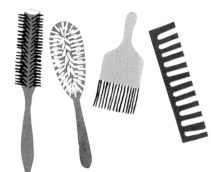

Styling products:

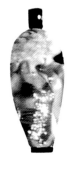

Shine control helps to tame frizzy curls and calm flyaway ends. A little goes a long way.

Gel provides a strong hold and gives a wet look when applied to damp hair.

Wax rubbed between your palms and smoothed over the surface of your hair will add shine and texture. You only need a tiny amount.

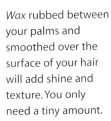

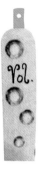

Volumising spray is spritzed on before styling. Concentrate on the roots of your hair to add lift and volume.

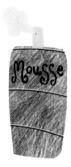

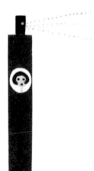

Mousse is one of the most popular styling products. Use on damp hair to give natural-looking lift and hold.

Hair spray should be used when all styling's done to hold your hard work in place.

Your dryer should be at least 1500 watts to cut down on drying time, but don't go too much higher or you could end up cooking your hair. Trading up? Invest in a dryer with a cool-air button as this instantly turns off the heating element to set your style and close cuticles to boost shine. The angle of your hair dryer is also important. Make sure it's pointing down so that the air blows your cuticles flat (and your hair shiny).

To straighten kinky hair or smooth out frizz, you need a large, round brush and a hair dryer with a cool-air button. Gently pat dry with a towel and apply a blow-dry lotion to protect your hair from the heat. Then clip back the top half, and working in small sections, move the brush through your hair with the dryer nozzle pointing downward. Make sure that the sections are completely dry before moving onto the next, and finish each one with a blast of cool air.

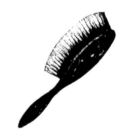

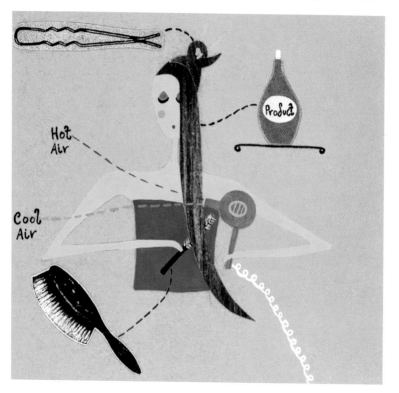

Hot Air

Cool Air

Product

65 Keep your hands out of your hair. The more you fuss, the flatter it will become as oil transfers from your hands.

66 Humidity is a frizzy hair horror. Smooth on a frizz-control lotion to coat the surface and repel outside moisture, and then stay out of steamy bathrooms (do your make-up in the bedroom instead).

67 Rub all styling products between your palms before smoothing over hair. That way you'll get an even distribution and won't risk overdoing it. Too much gunk and you'll end up with a greasy head.

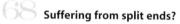

68 **Suffering from split ends?**
Apply leave-in conditioner to the
offending areas before using
heated appliances and your hair
will be protected from further
damage.

69 **A better way to blow in
volume** than hanging your head
upside down is to fling your hair
from side to side, lifting the roots
with a vent brush as you go.

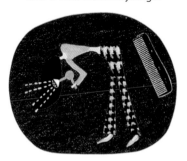

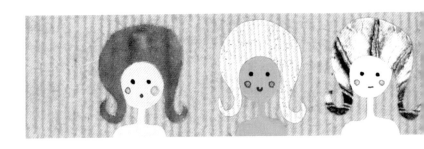

Every hair type needs its own help:

Oily hair needs washing daily with a mild shampoo. Avoid conditioner anywhere near the roots and swap your brush for a comb—which won't stimulate the oil glands.

Fine hair will look even finer if you have too many layers and too much length—a blunt cut is the best hair thickener money can buy.

Frizzy hair is best tamed by using a frizz-fighting lotion and being left to dry naturally.

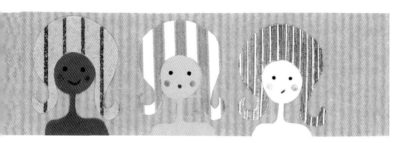

Dry hair should be kept well away from heated styling appliances, chemical treatments, the sun, and chlorinated swimming pools—all guaranteed to frazzle it more.

Dull hair can be refreshed by rinsing away any buildup of styling products with 2 tablespoons of white vinegar diluted in 1 cup of water after shampooing.

Limp hair should have light conditioner applied only to the very ends. Make sure that you rinse extra well afterward.

71 Curling Tools:

Heated rollers now come in hair-friendly rubber. If you own the old-fashioned spiky kind, place a piece of tissue around each one before winding to protect your hair.

Curling irons—use small irons for tight curls on short hair, use large irons for loose curls on long hair. Practice tucking in hair as "fishhook" ends will ruin your style. Don't hold the iron in your hair for too long.

Hot brushes are easier to use than curling irons because bristles hold the hair, but beware of tangles—it's easy for a hot brush to get lodged in your locks.

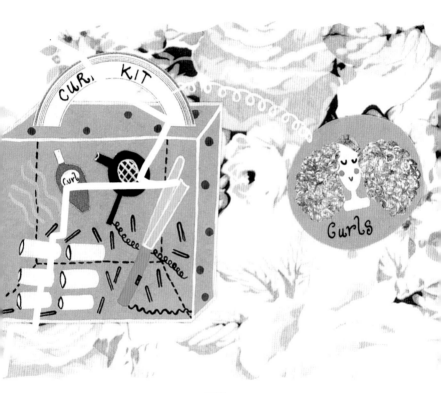

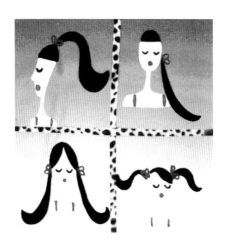

72 **Ponytail bands slip easily on shiny hair.** Use a piece of wet string instead. Tie it tightly and, as the string dries, it will contract to hold your hair firmly in place.

73 **Old bobby pins scratching your head?** No need to invest in a new package—simply dip the sharp ends in clear nail polish to seal the edges.

74 **Not just for fourth graders, braids are the choice of grown-up girls too.** Perfect for hiding hair overdue for washing. And if you braid your hair while it's still damp, the next day you'll be the proud owner of perfect waves. Far kinder than crimping.

75 **Tightly-curled hair is thin and twisty and needs gentle treatment to avoid tearing.** Not easy when the tiny curls wrap around each other, resulting in some serious tangles. But don't tug at them because stress to the roots can lead to hair loss. Excessive blow-drying, hot combing, and rollering are not going to help your delicate hair, so if straight's what you want, go for a chemical treatment instead. No chemicals are good for hair, but at least you'll be able to get a comb through it, and you won't need to go near a roller again. Straightening must be done by a professional and needs repeating every 12 to 16 weeks. Tightly-curled hair is the most vulnerable to damage so it needs moisturising products to keep it safe. And avoid sleeping in rollers or braiding too tightly—the main causes of hair falling out in clumps.

76 **If you're lucky enough to have thick, straight hair, you also have the strongest hair of all.** Not only that, it will probably grow faster than your friends' wavy hair. All those thick hairs mean natural body too, although many people with this hair type still have perms. If you are thinking about having a perm, consider that perms can cause serious damage as your strong hair will need a strong chemical to coax it

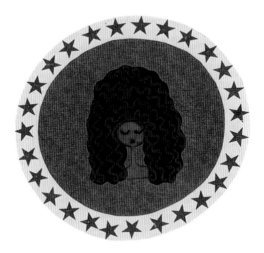

into curls. And with the shiniest type of hair, why not make the most of what you have and keep it straight and silky? But remember, if you grow it long, hair past shoulder length is more suscepti- ble to split ends. Use a deep conditioner and have a trim regu- larly. Always try to dry your hair naturally when possible—too much styling will eat away at those ends.

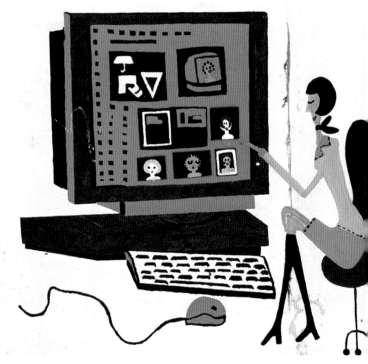

77 Late for work and running short on styling time? Rough dry your hair (by either patting it with a towel or using a hair dryer and your fingers) until it's just turning from wet to dry. That way any styling you do will get instantly locked in. Then concentrate on your hairline and the top of your head—the parts everyone sees.

78 For super sleek hair, slip a pair of panty hose over your hair, or tie a scarf around your head while you're applying your makeup. Having something tied tightly around your hair will help to smooth down cuticles and give you shiny hair without the styling.

79 For a quick fix for flat hair, spray it with a little water and then gently but firmly rub your palms over your head in large circles. This will lift the roots back up and help to re-introduce some body.

80 Suffering from static? A simple solution for hair that has a life of its own is to gently rub a fabric softener sheet over the surface. This should help to calm things down right away.

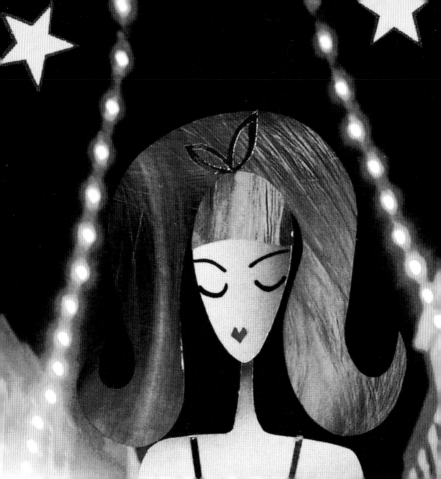

chapter 5

Sexy hair

Long blonde hair is the ultimate sexy style. Before bleach, you had to be born blonde, but then icons like Marilyn Monroe, Jean Harlow, and Mae West took to the bottle and inspired ordinary women to stand out from the crowd. Brigitte Bardot made a few films as a brunette, then decided to go blonde and became the archetypal "blonde bombshell" for thousands to follow. Blondes may not necessarily have more fun, but the right shade of blonde is always flattering. But don't try to bleach at home—a head full of straw won't cut it.

82 **Glitter in your hair is a sexy look for a special occasion.** Loose glitter is easier to use than spray, because you can sprinkle on as little, or as much, as you want. Spray glitter is less subtle as it will just cover whatever hair is in front of the nozzle. For the perfect look, finish styling and use hair spray, then sprinkle your glitter straight away so it sticks to the drying spray.

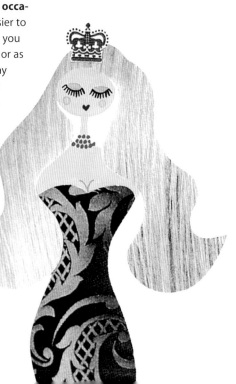

83 **Freshly washed hair smells best,** but if you're a long way from a shower, a squirt of perfume will do. Spray into the air, close your eyes and walk through the mist. It's also a good way to wear perfume if your nose likes the smell but your sensitive skin can't take it.

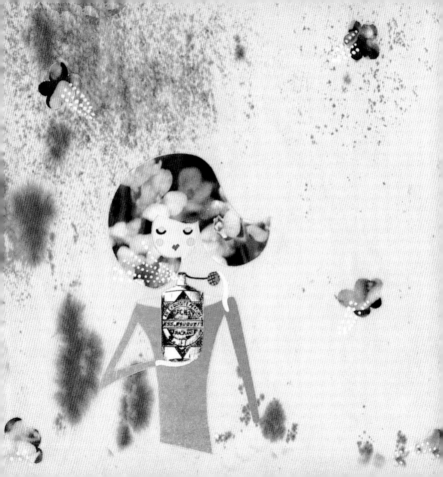

Hair that's spent a day on the beach looks great—and feels terrible. Get the tousled look minus the torture with a little help from a bottle of dry shampoo. Photographers' stylists swear by it for achieving that matte texture with lots of body (think salt water baked into your hair after a swim). Dry shampoo also gets you a day or two longer out of your blow-dry since it works best on hair that's a bit past its best. Shake the can well, and hold about 12 inches away from your hair as you puff it in. Work the powder through your roots using your hands to massage in volume. A quick shake and—Wow!—you're a beach babe.

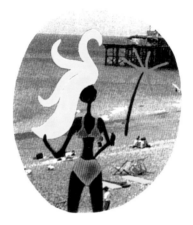

85 **Flat hair is never where it's at.** To revive yours, tip your head upside down and brush your hair in all different directions for extra lift. Then squirt hair spray into the roots, hold still for a second while it dries, and fling your head back over. The result? Instant body.

86 **Wear your hair in a bun on top of your head as the ultimate fix for a bad hair day.** Turn upside down and spritz with hair spray. Use a large brush to gather your hair into a high ponytail, wrap the end around, and secure with bobby pins.

Flips are cutesy, girly and always in fashion. Blow-dry yours in with the help of a round brush, but start styling only when your hair's almost dry or you'll be wasting precious getting-ready time. You can use a curling iron or a hot brush on already-dry hair to flip up those ends. Easy, fast, and you can even do the back yourself. For staying power, squirt a little hair spray on to your brush before the final flip.

Heading out on a hot date? Then take it easy with the hair spray. Men like hair that looks touchable, as if they could run their fingers through it. Hair that's stuck together like rock is not going to tempt his wandering hands. So for once, less is more. Use a body-building product before blow-drying to pump up the volume, then ruffle with your hands and leave your hair to do what comes naturally. He'll be yours for the taking!

Tinted hair polish is the newest way to add sexy color and shine. Just scoop a little up, rub between your palms, and then smooth over your hair's surface. As it catches the light, the color will too.

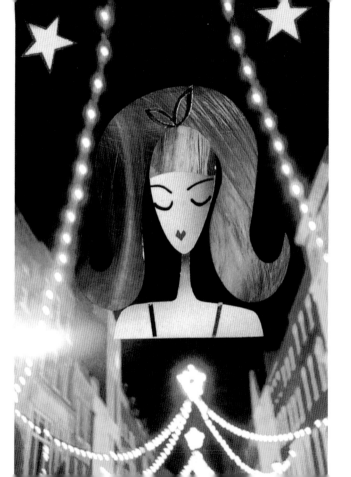

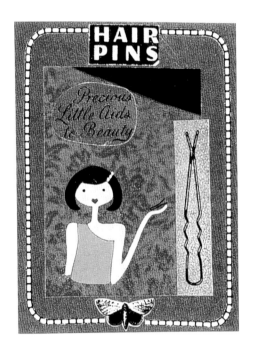

102

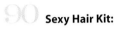

90 **Sexy Hair Kit:**

- *glittery barettes*
- *scrunchies*
- *hairpins*
- *covered bands*
- *tortoiseshell combs*
- *satin ribbons*
- *bobby pins*

A chignon is the classic way to wear long hair for a special occasion. When you can't make it to the hair salon, here's how to create the look at home.

What you need:

- *bobby pins*
- *hairpins*
- *a mirror to see the back of your head (or a helpful friend)*

What to do:

1. Brush all your hair to one side. Starting at the nape of your neck, put in a line of bobby pins right up the center back of your head, finishing just below the crown.

2. Working from the opposite side, carefully brush your loose hair back over the pins and then gently roll it into a long sausage shape directly over the line of bobby pins.

3. Use hairpins to secure your roll, sliding them under the bobby pins for an unmovable style.

4. Smooth any flyaway ends and then spritz with hair spray to hold all your hard work in place.

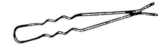

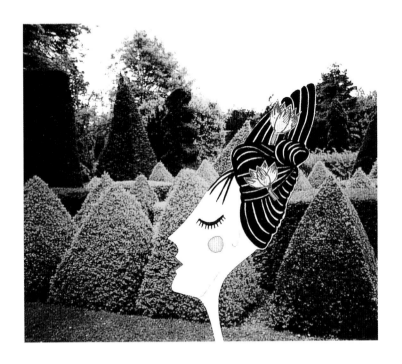

105

92 Crimping comes and goes, but there's no better way for making your hair look twice its size. Attempting to crimp your whole head yourself is time consuming and tricky (expect a dead arm after 20 minutes of mastering a heavy curling iron). A much easier method is to take random sections throughout your hair and crimp each one, starting at the roots and working down to the ends. Hold the curling iron tight for a few seconds and no longer before moving on, or the steam will start to rise. Then take a section of hair around your part and crimp the top hair so you look like you've done it all. For hair-friendly frizz, sleeping in braids will give you waves without the heat damage.

93 For a while, perms were out of it. That was until more modern techniques could give you waves without having them look like a wig. Make sure your hair's in top condition by giving it weekly deep-conditioning treatments for a month before you have a perm. Always allow at least a week between perming and coloring your hair, and don't be tempted to perm too often. As your roots start to droop, ask your hairdresser for a spot perm or wait until all your curls are gone before having another one. Perming on top of a perm equals frizz.

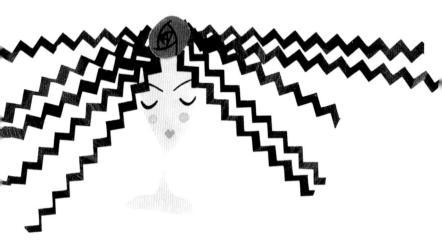

94 **Soft, face-framing waves are sexy and flattering.** To create them at home, comb styling gel through dry hair and make pin curls. Take small sections and twist them tightly so they coil back onto themselves. Pin securely. When your hair is completely dry, remove the pins and gently rake through with your fingers.

Hate your hair or just bored with what you've got? Wigs and hairpieces have come a long way since the "helmet hair" of years ago, and some top stylists now even produce their own lines. The right fit is everything. Too small and you'll end every day with a headache. Too large and you'll lose your new look on the dance floor. Look in the phone book for your local supplier and go for a fitting if you can. You can also order by phone from a mail-order catalog and experiment with new looks in the privacy of your home. Modern wigs are made with easy-to-style synthetic hair. Wash, shake, and drip dry. If only real hair were so easy.

A hairpiece can be your hair's best friend. Simply clip one on for added length and body to any style. But make sure you choose a piece that matches your own hair in color and texture. Too high a shine and you'll look like a Barbie doll. Take along your clip-on hairpiece to the salon when you go for a restyle and get your hairdresser to cut/dye it. Then no one will know where your hair ends and your hairpiece begins.

Ever wondered how celebrities go from short to long hair in a matter of weeks? The answer is hair extensions. That supermodel's hair you so admire? The chances are she's had a few fake strands put in to boost its body. Modern hair extensions are made of monofil, which is heat bonded to your own hair near the roots so the join is invisible. They will last up to four months, but you can take them out at any time, without damaging your own hair, by simply snapping the seal.

Once your extensions are in place, you can wash, brush, and style just as you always do, and your own hair will continue to grow without loosening the stuff on top. Most heads will only need a scattering of strands to add completely natural-looking body, lift, and length.

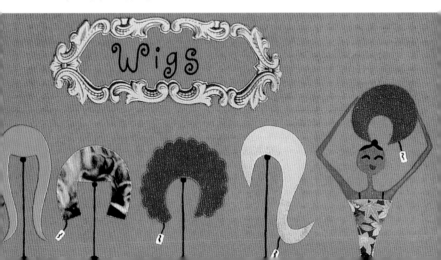

Wigs

There's nothing more glamorous than an "up do," but if your hair falls flat, take a tip from the '60s and relearn the art of the beehive. Back-combing has been replaced with back-brushing as the hair-friendly way to achieve all that flattering '60s height. Take sections of hair and gently push back the underneath strands toward the roots. Smooth the surface, tuck the ends under and pin in place.

A bouncy, poufy ponytail will always look more sexy than a slick, severe one. To create the look, set your hair in rollers before gathering it up and securing it with a pretty hair band.

Three simple but effective ways to get a perfect "up do."

1. Secure your hair in a covered elastic band. Pull your hair through the band once and then again, bringing your ponytail only halfway through. Tease out the ends with wax so they're sticking away from your head.

2. Hang your head upside down and pull your hair into a ponytail. Wind the tail around a band and secure with bobby pins.

3. Pull your hair into a low ponytail at the nape of your neck, twist it up the back of your head toward the crown and secure.

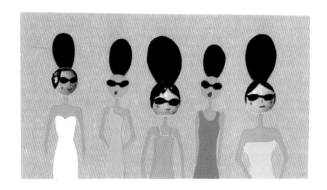

Copyright © MQ Publications Ltd 2000

Text © Liz Wilde 2000
Illustrations © Carol Morley 2000
Cover design: Broadbase
Interior Design: The Big Idea
Series Editor: Elizabeth Carr

Time Warner Books are published by
Time Warner Trade Publishing
1271 Ave. of the Americas
New York, NY 10020

Visit our Web site at www.twbookmark.com

For information on Time Warner Trade Publishing's online publishing
program, visit www.ipublish.com

 An AOL Time Warner Company

Printed in China
First printing: 10 9 8 7 6 5 4 3 2

Library of Congress Control Number: 2001094927

ISBN: 1-931722-01-3